A CONCISE SUMMARY OF **DAVID ZINC**

AND PETER MOORE'S

The 8 Hour Diet

...in 30 minutes

A 30 MINUTE HEALTH SUMMARY

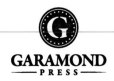

GARAMOND
——— P R E S S ———

CONTENTS

INTRODUCTION

Overview

Best-selling author and editor of *Men's Health* magazine David Zinczenko maintains that much of what people thought they knew about weight loss was wrong. Tapping into the research of leading experts on health and wellness, he has devised a diet plan that works on the cellular level and is based on restricting *when* a person eats rather than *what* a person eats. The results of following his 8-Hour Diet include a leaner, healthier body, an increase in energy, and a sharper mind.

Conventional weight-loss programs generally involve some kind of food restriction and a strict daily regimen. While they may work for a while, most people find it difficult to adhere to them over time. The 8-Hour Diet is easy to stick to because it allows people to eat anything they want—as long as they consume it within an eight-hour window.

As simple as that sounds, the plan devised by Zinczenko and his coauthor, Peter Moore, provides the context and structure essential for success. Citing numerous nutritional studies as background, they go on to offer a list of foods to include in those eight hours in order to maintain optimum health. And to help make sure those foods are easily incorporated into a meal plan, they provide easy-to-prepare recipes and an example of what a typical week on the diet might look like.

Exercise is strongly recommended here, but the exercise program they propose can be accomplished in as little as eight minutes per day. Suggested exercises are provided and explained step by step.

Perhaps the best news of all for anyone embarking on this program is the fact that it doesn't require a day-in, day-out commitment. The 8-Hour Diet works even if followed only three or four days a week—so there's no need to feel guilty or defeated when real-life social commitments or irresistible temptation get in the way of health and fitness.

In short, by making simple changes in daily eating patterns, people can train their bodies to operate more efficiently, burn fat, and even age more slowly.

About the Authors

David Zinczenko is the editor-in-chief of *Men's Health* magazine and the *New York Times* best-selling author of many books about diet and nutrition, including twelve books in the *Eat This, Not That* series and three books in the *Abs Diet* series. He is also the editorial director of *Women's Health, Prevention,* and *Organic Gardening* magazines. He has advocated for legislation declaring a national Men's Health Week and appears regularly on television talk shows to promote good health and weight loss.

Peter Moore is the coauthor of the *New York Times* best seller *The Lean Belly Prescription* and an editor at *Men's Health* magazine. He is the winner of a National Magazine Award.

How the Book Came About

As the editor of *Men's Health* and the author of many weight-loss books, Zinczenko has long been interested in finding ways to fight the national obesity epidemic with a simple, sustainable weight-loss program. When his father died of a stroke in 1999, he realized that his own hard-driving lifestyle needed to change. He began seeking a way to sustain a healthful weight that didn't involve exhausting daily workouts. He also needed a program that would allow him the flexibility to dine out with clients and authors without worrying about breaking his diet.

He began reviewing studies that showed the effectiveness of what is called *intermittent fasting,* and after trying it with much success, developed the plan he presents in *The 8-Hour Diet.* Published in December 2012, the book has won praise from commentators on a variety of national television shows, including *Today,* and in other media, including Boston.com.

THE GROUNDBREAKING SCIENCE BEHIND THE 8-HOUR DIET

Overview

This program isn't just about losing weight. Reducing the risk of disease and slowing down the aging process are benefits of the 8-Hour Diet as well. According to the authors, by fasting for sixteen hours a day, people's bodies are given a chance to rejuvenate and rid themselves of toxins. If people skip late-night snacks and exercise briefly in the morning instead of eating breakfast, their fat stores will burn away. They'll lose weight rapidly while enjoying an eight-hour window in which to eat more or less freely.

While regular, strenuous exercise is good for the body,
it is not necessary when following the 8-Hour Diet.
A simple, eight-minute workout is all that's
needed to jump-start the metabolism.

Chapter Summary

The 8-Hour Diet challenges the commonly held belief that breakfast is the most important meal of the day. In fact, says Zinczenko, eating first thing in the morning allows fat and toxins from the previous day's meals to remain stored and unused, promoting weight gain, aging, and disease. Skipping breakfast and waiting until late morning to have the first meal allows the body's mitochondria (tiny organs within cells) to dispose of the free radicals—responsible for aging and disease—produced as a byproduct of the energy they generate. When the previous day's food has time to break down properly before it is replaced, the mitochondria can do their work more efficiently.

In addition, the body stores fat that can be difficult to get rid of. When people skip the morning meal, their bodies begins to burn that stored fat. If they start the day with some light to moderate exercise, they jump-start the fat-burning process, and weight loss is accelerated. By foregoing late-night snacking, people continue to burn stored fat for fuel throughout the night, further increasing the value of the morning's exercise. By the time the first meal is consumed (the authors suggest 11:00 a.m. or later), people's bodies have had a chance to use the previous day's fuel as efficiently as possible.

Regularly eating foods that are high in fiber, protein, healthful fats, vitamins, and minerals promotes rapid weight loss, long-term health, and overall well-being. Then, not-so-healthful food can be consumed on occasion, with far less guilt.

Chapter 1: Key Points

- Cells in the body need time to burn all of the nutrients and toxins consumed the previous day. Withholding food for sixteen hours at a time is the most effective way to ensure that this happens efficiently.

- Fat stores itself predominantly in the abdominal area and can be very difficult to get rid of. *Intermittent fasting* jump-starts the body's use of this fat for fuel.

- By eating the final meal in the early evening and exercising in the morning, prior to the first one, the body's cells are allowed to "scrub" themselves of toxins and promote fat-burning. The results are rapid weight loss and an improvement in general health and well-being.

2

HOW THE 8-HOUR DIET
WILL CHANGE YOUR BODY

Overview

The human body is programmed to interact with the natural world, including the daily cycle of light and dark. Electricity has interrupted people's response to that cycle, allowing humans to be more active during the night. Much of people's nighttime activity includes eating, and this has contributed to the epidemic of obesity America is experiencing. Extra weight increases the risk of diabetes, heart disease, and cancer. Intermittent fasting allows the cells to detoxify and stored fat to burn as fuel. As pounds disappear, overall health risks decrease as well.

Research has demonstrated that people who eat a lot of fatty foods tend to eat more frequently throughout the day. By sticking to a balanced diet of healthful foods, the compulsion to eat is reduced and the weight comes off.

Chapter Summary

Throughout most of human history, the sun determined the level of human activity. With the invention of artificial light, people began to stay up well past sunset, and eating became an around-the-clock activity. Zinczenko considers this a contributing factor to the obesity epidemic and outlines the wide range of health problems associated with carrying excess weight—notably diabetes, heart disease, and cancer.

This chapter addresses the ways in which the 8-Hour Diet can help alleviate illnesses and conditions associated with obesity.

- Diabetes hampers the body's ability to produce and manage insulin. It is exacerbated by obesity and treated by restricting the consumption of foods high in sugar and fat. The risk of diabetes can be lessened, and the treatment of it can be aided, by adopting the intermittent fasting regimen of the 8-Hour Diet. When the body burns its fuel more efficiently, this includes the excess sugars associated with diabetes.

- Intermittent fasting can also reduce inflammation and bring down high cholesterol. Again, this is due to the increased efficiency of cell cleansing that occurs. The diet also promotes a rise in "good" cholesterol and lowers the level of triglycerides in the blood. All of this contributes significantly to a lower risk of heart disease.

- When cell growth is out of control, cancer occurs. It is well documented that diet contributes to at least some of the risk factors associated with cancer. Zinczenko maintains that reducing the amount of time during which the body receives fuel to stimulate cell growth reduces the risk of cancer.

The author points out that it is also important to get enough sleep, since the hormone melatonin is produced when darkness falls. Melatonin helps detoxify cells and works to help repair the body during sleep. But when natural nighttime drowsiness is counteracted by stimulation, melatonin production stops and so do its benefits.

People are more likely to get enough sleep when they go to bed and get up at around the same time every day, avoid drinking caffeine after 2:00 p.m., and forego exercise after the late afternoon. A hot bath prior to bedtime and a cool bedroom also aid in falling and staying asleep.

Chapter 2: Key Points

- The invention of electric light has disrupted the natural day-night cycle and opened the door to eating day and night. Just because people can doesn't mean they should!

- Fasting for sixteen hours per day allows people's bodies to cleanse themselves and burn their fat stores, helping everyone stay at a healthful weight and lessening the risks of diabetes, heart disease, and cancer associated with obesity.

- Getting sufficient sleep facilitates production of the hormone melatonin, which further repairs the body and promotes good health.

3

LONGER LIFE, STRONGER MIND

Overview

A lean, healthy body is not much good without a well-functioning mind.
Fortunately, according to Zinczenko, the physical results of the 8-Hour
Diet lead to a healthier mental state as well. Fasting promotes growth
and cleansing in nerve cells as well as muscle cells. Plus, by reducing
inflammation and levels of the hormone cortisol—produced when
people experience stress—the program helps guard against brain-based
diseases such as Alzheimer's, Parkinson's, and Huntington's. So...
thinner *and* smarter is the promise of this program.

---

*Try to exercise within the first half hour after waking up to
promote the maximum burning of fat stores. A brisk walk in
daylight is a great way to help maintain the body's
natural biorhythms.*

Chapter Summary

In addition to benefiting physical health, intermittent fasting is good for
mental health as well. To explain, the author focuses on a time when
life was lived during the daylight hours and humans were in constant
search of food.

As it did for early humans, fasting puts people into *hunting mode*—more alert, with heightened senses and energy reserves burning. But nowadays, people are rarely in hunting mode. They are far more likely to sit for most of the day, eat three large meals, and reach for snacks in between them. This leaves people obese, unhealthy, and with a distinct lack of mental acuity.

A study by the Institute of Aging affirms that fasting promotes the production of proteins called *neurotropic factors* that strengthen the mind and help protect it from Alzheimer's, Huntington's, and Parkinson's diseases. The implication is that nerve cells receive the same benefits from intermittent fasting that muscle cells do.

The brain requires more energy than any other organ and responds to fasting just as muscles do, creating more cells and links among cells when stressed by lack of fuel. And brain cells sweep out toxins and other detritus just as muscle cells do.

Fasting for sixteen hours per day has been shown to:

- Reduce inflammation throughout the body—including in the brain—helping combat the onset of Alzheimer's disease.

- Reduce levels of the hormone cortisol, which directs the body to store fat.

- Reduce the incidence of stroke by clearing blood vessels throughout the body, including in the brain.

- Promote *neuroplasticity*, the brain's ability to renew and regenerate itself, even as the body ages.

- Encourage the manufacture of new cells in the hippocampus, the portion of the brain responsible for memory.

Adopting a lifestyle closer to that of human's early ancestors by fasting and exercising regularly is beneficial to both people's bodies and people's minds.

A mid-afternoon nap is a much better option for revitalizing the body than a sugary snack. Around 2:00 p.m., try to find a quiet place and catch a fifteen- or twenty-minute snooze to feel rejuvenated throughout the afternoon and evening.

Chapter 3: Key Points

- The brain functions at its highest level when a person is hungry and in *hunting mode*—so fasting keeps a person sharp and focused.

- By reducing inflammation, stress, and other brain-damaging factors, intermittent fasting helps reduce the chances of stroke and a variety of brain diseases.

- Fasting promotes the generation of new cells, keeping people's brains healthy and growing throughout a lifetime.

FAST QUESTIONS, FAST ANSWERS

Overview

While the concept of the 8-Hour Diet is easy to grasp, questions can arise in the course of following it. In this chapter, the author anticipates and answers such questions as: Must I fast during the same period every day? Can I really eat anything I want? Is this a good program for a competitive athlete? Will the diet work for vegetarians? Is it possible to take breaks during the week?

Since this program is designed to accommodate people who lead busy lives and need flexibility, all of these questions have "good news" answers.

It is possible to go off the 8-Hour Diet for up to four days and still lose weight. However, it is a good idea to try to eat as sensibly as possible on "off days."

Chapter Summary

Here are some answers to the most frequently asked questions about the 8-Hour Diet.

- It isn't necessary to fast during the same sixteen-hour period each day.

- The plan works if it's followed for as few as three days per week—and they don't have to be three consecutive days.

- Yes, people really can eat anything they want during the eight-hour period.

- Coffee and tea are allowed during the fasting period, and even a small amount of milk or cream is permissible—but it is best to stick to water and sugar-free drinks.

- The 8-Hour Diet works fine for athletes and those who work out regularly.

- If hungry during the fasting period, drink something instead of giving in to the temptation to eat, or try distractions, such as taking a walk or engaging in a conversation.

- Try to eat a sensible amount during the eight-hour eating window.

- The diet accelerates the metabolism because fasting burns fat instead of muscle. That's why the results are likely to be better than what people experience on another kind of diet.

- It's fine for people to take their usual vitamins and supplements while following the 8-Hour Diet.

- The 8-Hour Diet is safe for vegetarians—but be sure to consume a healthful amount of protein during the eating window.

While it's true that people can eat anything they want during their eight-hour window, the program works best if people are mindful of eating a variety of foods from the eight suggested food groups. And try to keep meals and snacks moderate if possible.

Chapter 4: Key Points

- It's okay to go off the diet when necessary; it will still work if followed at least three days per week.

- The start and end times of the sixteen-hour fasting window can vary from one day to the next.

- Thirst can be mistaken for hunger and drinking can be a substitute for eating. Water and non-caloric drinks can satiate the appetite during the fasting period.

Bonus

TURN ANY DIET INTO AN 8-HOUR DIET

Overview

Incorporating the principles of intermittent fasting into other popular diet regimens can improve the results of those diets. There's a reason why Atkins, South Beach, and other diets are popular: they work for many people, the science is sound, and they are relatively easy to incorporate into daily living. But when users of any of those diets want to try a new program, they have to abandon the old one. Not so with the 8-Hour Diet, which can be used in conjunction with other programs. In fact, it might even be preferable to use the 8-Hour Diet along with another plan—since each can enhance the benefits of the other.

Chapter Summary

Here is a rundown of some popular diet plans with notes on how they can be combined with the 8-Hour Diet.

- **Atkins** is a high-protein diet. Incorporating intermittent fasting into Atkins can accelerate weight loss and help fend off chances of stroke and heart disease.

- **Paleo** rules out processed foods. It can be combined with the 8-Hour Diet—but adding dairy and whole grains can increase the overall benefits.
- **South Beach** is a modified high-protein plan similar to Atkins that includes grains, fruits, and vegetables. Intermittent fasting can enhance its benefits and pick up the pace of weight loss.
- **Wheat Belly** is heavy on protein, fats, nuts, and vegetables while restricting carbohydrates. Coupling it with intermittent fasting can help reduce the risk of diabetes.
- **New Abs**, developed by the author of *The 8-Hour Diet*, features low-fat foods combined with protein powder supplements. Adding intermittent fasting can lead to a faster six-pack.
- **Eat This, Not That** is Zinczenko's own survey of healthful convenience food options. Combining the information in it with the 8-Hour Diet can make intermittent fasting easier for any lifestyle.

Bonus Chapter: Key Points

- There are many popular diet plans out there and it is important each person chooses the one that works for them.

- The principles of the 8-Hour Diet can be incorporated into virtually any good diet program—and improve the results.

- Combining the 8-Hour Diet with another plan can help people stick to the diet they've chosen until they reach their goals.

5

THE 8 FOODS YOU SHOULD EAT EVERY DAY

Overview

Although one of the principles of the 8-Hour Diet is that there are no restrictions on food consumed within the window, the authors suggest users should incorporate items from eight food groups into their daily meal plan. These *8-Hour Powerfoods*, selected to maximize health, energy, and weight loss, include lean meats, eggs, nuts, yogurt and other dairy, beans, fruits, fresh greens, and whole grains.

When considering which fruits and vegetables to incorporate into a daily food plan, it's a good idea to mix as many colors as possible, since foods of each color have specific health benefits.

Chapter Summary

Although "anything goes" on this plan in terms of food choice and quantity, certain foods should be eaten regularly to maintain optimal health and maximize weight loss. Zinczenko calls these the 8-Hour Powerfoods and recommends that they be included in any daily food regimen.

Four of the food groups are called *Fat Busters* and consist of foods high in fiber, healthful fats, and protein. The other four are called *Health Boosters*, and they are rich in vitamins and minerals.

Fat Busters

- **Lean meats, eggs, and fish.** Foods such as tuna, salmon, and sardines are rich in Omega-3 fatty acids, which lowers a hormone that helps store body fat. Eggs are an excellent protein source and help build muscle.

- **Walnuts, almonds, sunflower seeds, and avocados.** Nuts are a great source of protein and monounsaturated fat, and help ease hunger.

- **Yogurt, low-fat milk, cheese, and cottage cheese.** Dairy strengthens bones, helps lower blood pressure, and aids in the breakdown of body fat.

- **Beans, legumes, and peanuts (including peanut butter).** These foods help prevent muscle loss, heart disease, colon cancer, high blood pressure, and wrinkles. They are also a great source of protein.

Health Boosters

- **Raspberries, strawberries, blueberries, and blackberries.** Berries are high in antioxidants, which help clean out cell toxins, as well as fiber, and salicylic acid, which help prevent blood clots.

- **Apples, oranges, watermelon, cantaloupe, and tomatoes.** These fruits are excellent sources of vitamin C and fiber, and help prevent heart disease and cancer.

- **Spinach, broccoli, asparagus, peppers, yellow and green beans, lettuces, mustard greens, and kale.** These and other greens are great sources of vitamins A, C, and K, fiber, and beta-carotene. Lettuces also help fend off heart disease and various cancers.

- **Whole grains and cereals, brown rice, whole-wheat pretzels, whole-wheat pastas, and quinoa.** These foods are great sources of fiber, thiamin, niacin, vitamin E, and more. They help prevent cancer, high blood pressure, and heart disease.

Olive oil is a healthful fat that lowers cholesterol, strengthens the immune system, helps the body burn fat, and helps control food cravings. Use it instead of transfats, margarine, or vegetable oil.

Chapter 5: Key Points

- Yes, people can eat anything they want in the eight-hour window, but a diet that is unbalanced or based on unhealthful foods is counterproductive.

- Including foods from all eight categories of the *8-Hour Powerfoods* will help ensure health, weight loss, and longevity.

- Though fresh foods are the most flavorful, there is nearly as much nutrition in frozen berries and spinach.

6

THE 8-HOUR SAMPLE EATING PLAN

Overview

The concept of eating within an eight-hour window is simple enough, but it is helpful to have a sense of what that looks like. To outline a typical day on the diet, Zinczenko asked a friend who follows the program to itemize her routine.

The 8-hour window can be adjusted each day, depending on each person's schedule. As long as the fasting period is sixteen consecutive hours, eating can begin whenever the day's activities demand.

Chapter Summary

Here's what a typical day on the 8-Hour Diet looks like.

7:00 a.m.:	Coffee and eight minutes of exercise.
10:30 a.m.:	Smoothie of berries, mango, yogurt, and orange juice.
11:30 a.m.:	Snack of hummus and pita chips.
1:00 p.m.:	Lunch of turkey sandwich on whole-wheat bread with cheese, guacamole, and bacon.
3:00 p.m.:	Snack of chips and salsa.

4:00 p.m.: Americano coffee (espresso and hot water).

6:00 p.m.: Dinner of sirloin burger with tossed green salad; scoop of ice cream sprinkled with nuts for dessert.

8:00 p.m.: Cup of tea with honey and low-fat milk.

Chapter 6: Key Points

- The only way to make a diet work is for people to change their habits and stick to the new ones until they are second nature. Once people get the hang of eating this way, they can do it for life.

- Doing at least eight minutes of exercise each morning promotes fat burning and staves off hunger until the first meal.

- Light snacking between meals (but only during the window!) can help keep energy from slumping—but reach for one of the 8-Hour Powerfoods if possible.

7

THE 8-HOUR DIET CHEAT PLAN

Overview

Many diets fail because they require strict adherence to the regimen in order to work. As with anything in life, people will get out of a diet only what they put in—but the 8-Hour Diet is unique in that people can "cheat" and still enjoy its benefits. In this chapter, the author provides a series of strategies to mitigate the damage when life imposes itself on one's best intentions. From drinking coffee or water to working out to making sure to get enough sleep, there are many effective forms of "damage control" people can employ. But even when the health program goes off the rails completely, the 8-Hour Diet program is a forgiving one.

When faced with a stressful situation such as an upcoming deadline, a major meeting, or some other significant event, try sticking to the intermittent fasting routine for several days beforehand. The mind-sharpening benefits can enhance one's performance.

Chapter Summary

Here are some things to remember when coping with the ups and downs of dieting.

Strategy #1: Going off and on the 8-Hour Diet isn't a problem, as long as people follow it three or more days a week. The fat-burning effects from just one day of intermittent fasting have been shown to last beyond a day.

Strategy #2: Hunger can often be assuaged by drinking liquid. Coffee is an excellent appetite suppressant, and putting a little milk in coffee or tea is acceptable.

Strategy #3: Distraction is a good way to fend off hunger. Going to a movie, exercising, or working late can help prevent eating during the fasting period.

Strategy #4: Going to bed earlier than usual can help prevent late-night snacking, and sleep has been shown to aid in weight loss.

Strategy #5: A round of vigorous exercise can replace a meal. Physical exertion is a great appetite killer.

Strategy #6: If people are going to have a "cheat meal," pick protein. A steak, a cheeseburger, or an omelet can help the body build muscle while it's burning fat. The best time to go heavy on protein is at the first meal of the day.

Strategy #7: Eat a majority of the day's carbohydrates at night. Studies have shown that the body burns carbs most efficiently at the end of the day.

Strategy #8: Plan each fasting day's meals and snacks ahead of time so as not to act on impulse when hungry.

Bonus Strategy: Food tends to taste better when the body has rested from eating for an extended period—making that first meal especially pleasurable, even if the portions are judicious. Enjoy each bite.

Intermittent fasting has been studied across several cultures and shown to promote good health. Mormons fast one day a month and Muslims fast (intermittently) one month a year. Whatever the religious significance, the physical benefits are clear.

Chapter 7: Key Points

• Most diets require 24/7 adherence to their rules to work. The fact that the 8-Hour Diet is more flexible makes it easier to adhere to over time.

• When people need to take a day off, curb the damage by using common-sense strategies, such as adding a workout, drinking to satisfy one's appetite, getting some extra sleep, and planning meals mindfully.

• Make nutritional science a friend: Consume protein early in the day and carbs at night.

8

THE 8-MINUTE RECIPES

Overview

One of the biggest attractions of the 8-Hour Diet is that no food is off-limits. It's even permissible to "cheat." But of course the plan works best when people stick with it and draw liberally from the eight food groups outlined in Chapter 5.

In this chapter, the author offers dozens of recipes for healthful breakfasts, lunches, dinners, and snacks, using many of the Fat Busters and Health Boosters he identified previously. Preparing these dishes—or coming up with unique variations using ingredients from the eight food groups—will ensure a well-nourished body. And when that's the case, people are less likely to cheat!

Breakfast tip: Use a whole-wheat frozen waffle as a base for an open-faced breakfast sandwich. Top it with scrambled eggs, turkey, and guacamole; cheese, strawberries, and agave syrup; or peanut butter, banana, sliced almonds, and honey.

Chapter Summary

Here is a sample of the dishes the author describes, most of which can be prepared in eight minutes or less.

Breakfast

- **Smoothies:** Use fruits or fruit juices, yogurt or milk, ground flaxseed, protein powder, mint, ginger, etc.
- **Sunrise Sandwich:** Fry egg in olive oil, microwave turkey and one slice of cheese thirty seconds, add tomato and guacamole, and layer on English muffin.
- **Waffles with Ham and Eggs:** Fry Canadian bacon and two eggs; toast waffles; top with meat, maple syrup, Cheddar cheese, and eggs.
- **Oatmeal with Peanut Butter and Banana:** Cook oatmeal for five minutes; add banana, peanut butter, chopped almonds, and agave syrup.

Lunch

- **Spinach and Ham Quiche:** Lightly bake frozen pie shell eight minutes; sauté garlic and spinach; mix ham, cheese, eggs, milk, half-and-half, spinach, salt, and nutmeg; pour into pie shell and bake for about twelve minutes.
- **Chinese Chicken Salad:** Slice Napa and red cabbage into thin strips; toss with sugar in a bowl; heat shredded chicken in microwave; toss chicken and cabbage with cilantro, Mandarin oranges, sliced almonds, and Asian-style vinaigrette.
- **Chicken Salad Sandwich with Raisins and Curry:** Soak raisins in hot water for ten minutes and drain; add chopped, cooked chicken, sliced celery, diced onion, shredded carrots, curry powder, and mayonnaise; spread on two slices of whole-grain bread or English muffin.

- **The Ultimate Burger:** Form chopped sirloin and brisket into four patties; cook for two to three minutes on each side; place on toasted hamburger buns with arugula and caramelized onions.

Dinner

- **Grilled Fish Tacos with Mango Salsa:** Mix mango, avocado, onion, cilantro, and lime juice; grill mahi-mahi fillet four minutes on each side; warm tortillas on the grill for one minute; break fish into chunks and arrange on tortilla; top with cabbage and mango salsa.
- **Honey-Mustard Salmon with Roasted Asparagus:** Toss asparagus with olive oil; mix butter and brown sugar in a bowl and microwave for thirty seconds; stir in mustard, honey, and soy sauce; rub salmon with the mixture, place on top of the asparagus, and roast in preheated oven at 450 degrees for eight to ten minutes; remove, brush with more honey-mustard, and top with sesame seeds.
- **Grilled Pork and Peaches:** Brush thick-cut pork chops with olive oil, grill four to five minutes per side; brush peach halves with oil and place on grill for five minutes; toss peaches with pine nuts, onion, blue cheese, and vinegar; top chops with mixture.
- **Super Supreme Pizza:** Cover the crust of a store-bought whole-wheat, thin-crust pizza shell with tomato-basil pasta sauce, cheese, pepperoni, onion, peppers, olives, garlic, pepper flakes, and artichokes; bake for twelve to fifteen minutes at 400 degrees; top with basil.

Snacks

- **Parmesan Roasted Broccoli:** Toss broccoli with olive oil, salt, and pepper; roast in 450 degree oven for twelve minutes; toss with Parmesan cheese.
- **Ultimate Guacamole:** Grind cilantro and garlic together into a fine paste; add to avocado and smash into puree; stir in onions, jalapeno, lemon juice, and salt.
- **Smoky Deviled Eggs:** Cook eggs for eight minutes in boiling water and peel when cool; cut in half and scoop out yolk; mix yolk with mayonnaise, mustard, chipotle, salt, and pepper; put in plastic bag with small hole in one corner, pipe the mixture into the egg-white halves; sprinkle with paprika and crumbled bacon.

Nonstick pans are great because they allow the use of less oil—but when they are overheated, they can release harmful chemicals. When using a nonstick pan, monitor the temperature carefully.

Chapter 8: Key Points

- Preparing food at home allows people to monitor more carefully the amount of fat, sugar, salt, and other ingredients taken in each day.

- Using fresh, non-processed foods promotes good health and weight loss.

- Many great meals can be prepared in as little as eight minutes.

9

CHANGE YOUR MIND
TO CHANGE YOUR BODY

Overview

People eat for a great many reasons in addition to hunger—boredom, anger, sadness, celebration, and more. Mindless eating is something everyone has experienced, and an excess of it can lead to obesity and poor health. Though this diet plan allows people to eat anything they want within an eight-hour window, temptation may strike when that window has closed (or overrule a person's good sense during eating hours). On the days when a fast is planned, it is helpful to have some distractions on hand to keep one's mind out of the kitchen.

Chapter Summary

When hunger strikes at an inopportune time, it's a good idea to seek distraction. Here are some useful ways to take one's mind off food.

- Watch a video.
- Finish a project that's been put off.
- Work off hunger in the gym.
- Tighten muscles when hunger strikes.
- Visualize eating.

- Call someone for support.
- At work, focus on tasks and avoid the candy jar.
- Breathe deeply.
- The color black is said to be an appetite suppressant; decorate the office accordingly.
- Browse through old photo albums.
- Play video games.
- Keep a journal.
- Silently repeat the reasons for dieting.
- Note how long it takes a craving to subside.
- Visualize saying no to temptation.
- Play word games.
- Talk about the program with a friend.
- Follow an established routine.
- Find inspiration in success.
- Stay out of the kitchen.
- Drink green or oolong tea; add cinnamon if preferred.
- Remember that prehistoric people went days without food.
- Wear fancier clothes.
- Write down the reasons for following the program.
- Drink water with fresh citrus juice or herbs.
- Drink peppermint tea.
- Set a goal.
- Drink yerba maté.
- Drink sparkly water.
- Take frequent, short walks.
- Add flavors to ice cubes before freezing.
- Drink black tea.
- Drink coffee.
- Go for a run.

- Go for a workout.
- Make vegetable stock.
- Take a nap.
- Do some light yoga.
- Play a sport.
- Walk the dog.
- Wash the car.
- Do some stretches.
- Ride a bike.
- Take up a hobby.
- Take a walk.
- Visit colleagues instead of emailing them.
- Smell food.
- Chew sugar-free gum.
- Chew ice.
- Light scented candles.
- Dance.
- Go out in the sun.
- Meditate.
- Brush and floss.
- Clean the toilet.
- Cuddle with someone.
- Get a massage.
- Have sex.
- Go to the spa.
- Thank someone.
- Learn a new song.
- Do the dishes.
- Be nice to someone.

Chapter 9: Key Points

- Hunger isn't always what it seems. There are many tricks and distractions for facing hunger during fasts.

- It helps to keep one's mouth busy with non-calorie beverages—or just talking.

- Dieting has a strong mental component. People should keep a positive attitude, remember why they are doing it, know that they are strong enough to avoid temptation— and forgive themselves if they succumb.

THE 8-MINUTE WORKOUTS

Overview

Exercise is an important component of any weight-loss program, and this one is no exception. The difference is that on this plan, eight minutes of exercise per day is all it takes to burn fat stores and accelerate weight loss. This chapter provides a number of fairly simple exercises that can be done in various combinations during each morning's eight-minute workout.

For maximum fat burning, exercises should be done shortly after waking. This accelerates the process by which the body builds muscle and processes the energy of the food consumed the day before.

Chapter Summary

One-Exercise Routines

Don't overstrain yourself if you don't regularly exercise. A beginner's goal is to burn calories and deplete the body's glycogen stores. Choose one exercise and continue the movement for eight minutes.

- **Jogging.** Option 1: Steady pace. Option 2: Alternate slow and fast.
- **Running in Place.** Alternate running hard for sixty seconds and resting for sixty seconds.
- **Burpees.** Bending at hips and knees, lower body into a squat; place palms on a box six to twelve inches high; kick legs backward; jump legs back into squat; quickly stand up. Repeat.
- **Alternating Reverse Lunges.** Standing up straight, step back with left foot; lower body and bend front knee 90 degrees; return to standing position. Do the same with other leg. Repeat.

Two-Exercise Routines

Do eight reps of one exercise, then eight reps of another exercise for eight minutes.

- **Mountain Climber.** In a push-up position, lift right foot and move toward chest, then return to starting position. Repeat with left leg. Alternate quickly.
- **Body-Weight Power Squat.** Standing with feet slightly more than shoulder-width apart, push hips back and swing arms backward, lowering body; pause and return to start; swing arms above the head and stand on toes. Repeat.
- **Bucking Hop.** With hands and knees on the floor, raise knees off the floor; hop feet off the floor to the right, then to the left. Repeat.
- **Alternating Lateral Lunge.** With feet hip-width apart, take step to the left, bend left knee, and lower the body over it; return to starting position; repeat with right leg.

- **Push-up Hold with Knee-Elbow Touch.** In standard push-up position, lift right foot, bend knee, and try to touch knee with right elbow; return to starting position; repeat with left leg. Continue to alternate.
- **T-Rotation.** In standard push-up position, lift right hand and turn right side of body up until facing sideways and forming a T; return to start and repeat on left side. Continue to alternate.

Combined Exercise Intervals

Do one exercise for sixty seconds, followed by another one immediately. Rest one minute and do a second round.

- **Hip Extension.** Lie on back, knees bent and feet flat. With arms at an angle to the sides, palms down, raise hips to straighten body shoulder to knees; hold for two seconds; return to start. Repeat.
- **Push-up with Leg Lift.** In push-up position, lift right foot off the ground and do a push-up; return and repeat with left leg. Continue to alternate.
- **Body-Weight Rotational Squat.** Standing with feet shoulder-width apart, push hips back and bend knees to lower body; push back to starting position while pivoting feet and rotating torso to the right; repeat the movement, this time rotating to the left on the way up. Continue to alternate.

People who have not exercised regularly should not attempt to become body builders overnight. There is value even in mild exercise. An eight-minute walk around the neighborhood is a good way to start an exercise program.

Chapter 10: Key Points

- Exercise is important not only for weight loss but for overall health and well-being.

- It doesn't take a rigorous or time-consuming daily regimen to enjoy the effects of exercise; a brisk walk or eight minutes of moderate movement is beneficial.

- By exercising in the morning, the fat-burning and muscle-building mechanisms of the body are maximized.

CONCLUSION

Losing weight is not difficult—many weight-loss programs are effective. But the 8-Hour Diet is designed with enough flexibility to adapt to real-world situations, so it is easy to follow and easy to stay with until goals are met.

By skipping breakfast and starting the day with some mild (or vigorous) exercise, a person's body is given the chance to metabolize the food consumed the day before, burning fat and toxins more efficiently. This approach is so effective that it works well when practiced as little as three times a week—and combines well with other diet plans, too.

Within the eight-hour eating window, any kind of food can be consumed in any amount, but for maximum effectiveness, a common-sense approach is best. The eight food groups identified here—four groups of Fat Busters and four groups of Health Boosters—should be added to the menu on a daily basis in order to optimize weight loss and good health. These include lean meat, fresh vegetables, fruits, nuts, and dairy.

There is room for indulgence on the 8-Hour Diet, as long as everything is consumed within the eight-hour window. Drinking plenty of water, getting lots of sleep, and devising other distractions when necessary should help stave off temptation during the sixteen-hour fasting period. On the 8-Hour Diet, weight loss can be achieved relatively quickly and sustained over time.

Lightning Source UK Ltd.
Milton Keynes UK
UKOW041815230513

211184UK00001B/110/P